ADRENAL FATIGUE

Regain Energy and *Relieve* Your Stress

Sorrel Davis

live healthy now!

Healthy Living Publications
Summertown, Tennessee

Cover and interior design: Scattaregia Design

Book Publishing Company
PO Box 99
Summertown, TN 38483
888-260-8458
bookpubco.com

ISBN: 978-1-57067-374-0

Disclaimer
The information in this book is presented for educational purposes only. It isn't intended to be a substitute for the medical advice of a physician, dietitian, or other health-care professional.

Printed in the United States of America

24 23 22 21 20 19 1 2 3 4 5 6 7 8 9

Library of Congress Cataloging-in-Publication Data

Names: Davis, Sorrel, author.
Title: Adrenal fatigue : regain energy and relieve your stress / Sorrel Davis.
Description: Summertown, Tennessee : Healthy Living Publications, [2019]
Identifiers: LCCN 2019002736 | ISBN 9781570673740 (pbk.)
Subjects: LCSH: Adrenal glands--Diseases--Treatment--Popular works. | Fatigue--Treatment--Popular works. | Self-care, Health--Popular works.
Classification: LCC RC659 .D378 2019 | DDC 616.4/5--dc23
LC record available at https://lccn.loc.gov/2019002736

We chose to print this title on responsibly harvested paper stock certified by the Forest Stewardship Council, an independent auditor of responsible forestry practices. For more information, visit https://us.fsc.org.

MIX
Paper from responsible sources
FSC www.fsc.org FSC® C005010

CONTENTS

Introduction

In 1998 James L. Wilson coined the term "adrenal fatigue" to identify a condition that he believes is the consequence of ongoing stress: below-optimal adrenal function. He devised this term to put a name to the cluster of common symptoms that he asserts are caused by modern stress and to distinguish it from Addison's disease, a serious, long-term endocrine disorder. But many doctors say these symptoms can be due to other health problems or that the "symptoms" are merely very common complaints experienced by people in general.

Who is right? Is adrenal fatigue a true medical condition, or is it something simply construed by a well-meaning but misguided individual? Is it physiologically possible for the adrenal glands to malfunction or become depleted due to excessive stress? What tests are available to confirm a diagnosis of "adrenal fatigue"? And what treatment methods are medically endorsed and scientifically proven to alleviate the symptoms associated with it? The answers to these questions and more are explored in the following pages.

The Birth of "Adrenal Fatigue"

Ever since James Wilson first coined the term "adrenal fatigue," it has been widely employed by alternative health-care providers to describe an alleged condition caused by chronic exposure to stressful situations. The body's reactions to stress are associated with an enhanced secretion of a number of hormones, such as adrenaline and cortisol, that increase the mobilization of energy sources and adapt the individual to its new circumstance. The adrenal glands—small organs located above the kidneys—help the body cope with stress by producing these so-called stress hormones.

Supporters of the concept of adrenal fatigue believe the condition begins when the various stressors of life overwhelm the body and become too much for it to handle. According to the theory behind adrenal fatigue, when people are confronted with ongoing stress for long periods of time, their adrenal glands are unable to keep up with the body's demand for these stress hormones. When that occurs, symptoms of "adrenal fatigue" begin to surface.

Wilson not only conceived the term for the disorder, but he also invented exclusive diagnosis and treatment protocols, positioning himself as the premiere expert, diagnostician, and practitioner to both identify and cure the condition. In addition, Wilson developed specific tests and supplements, as well as an education and training program for other practitioners of his protocols who are eligible for wholesale supplement discounts, clinical support, and patient referrals. Despite the fact that Wilson's protocols have no medical endorsement or scientific proof, his theories and methods have proliferated worldwide.

Stress: The "Disease" of the 21st Century

Because stress is at the heart of supposed adrenal fatigue, any discussion pertaining to it must begin with a basic understanding of stress and the stress-coping mechanisms of the body. Everybody knows what stress is, or they think they do, since we've all experienced it at one time or another. Stress is basically an unavoidable consequence of contemporary life, and it could justifiably be deemed the "disease" of the twenty-first century. Although we all have encountered stress, most people would be hard pressed to define exactly what it is.

At its core, stress is a physiological (condition of the body) state with psychological (mental/emotional) components that is produced by a change in the environment (that is, a stressor) that disrupts the body's internal balance known as physiological homeostasis. Generally speaking, "stress" could be described as any situation that tends to disturb the equilibrium between a living organism and its environment.

Trying to Define the Elusive

Because the experience of stress is highly subjective, it's almost impossible to define it within a medical framework. If a medical phenomenon can't be accurately defined, it also can't be accurately measured. And if it can't be accurately measured, it can't be quantified, which makes it a challenge to observe and research it scientifically.

Complicating matters further is the fact that stress can be both positive and healthy (eustress)—as occurs with favorable situations, such as getting married, starting a new job, or buying a house—or negative and harmful (distress), which is how we most commonly define it. In addition, what one person perceives as a stressful event may be exciting or even dull to another person depending on a variety of uniquely individual factors, such as personality, physical strength, age, gender, life experiences, genetic makeup, or general health.

The Physiological Effects of Stress

While it's fairly obvious that excessive stress can negatively affect coping skills and impair a person's ability to manage the activities of daily living, the effect stress has on the various systems, organs, and tissues of the body is less apparent but equally significant. The following list shows how some of the key body systems respond to stress:

Nervous system. When the body is under stress, the sympathetic nervous system activates the fight-or-flight response. This triggers the release of "stress hormones," such as adrenaline and cortisol, from the adrenal glands. These hormones elevate heart rate, raise blood pressure, increase blood glucose levels, and interfere with digestive processes.

Musculoskeletal system. When the body is under stress, muscles tense and become more rigid, potentially triggering headaches, neck and back pain, and a variety of musculoskeletal problems.

Respiratory system. Stress can cause hyperventilation, which may lead to abnormal loss of carbon dioxide from the blood and which in turn can trigger panic attacks.

Cardiovascular system. Stress that's extreme but temporary causes an increase in heart rate, stronger contractions of the heart muscle, and the dilation of blood vessels that direct blood to the heart. Repeated episodes can inflame coronary arteries and may contribute to heart attacks.

Endocrine system. When the body is under stress, the brain sends signals from the hypothalamus to the adrenal glands to produce epinephrine, which triggers the liver to produce more glucose.

Gastrointestinal system. Stress can cause heartburn or acid reflux and, in extreme cases, nausea and vomiting. It can impair nutrient absorption and digestion and may trigger either constipation or diarrhea. It can also cause a loss of appetite or provoke overeating.

Reproductive system. Stress can induce irregular menstrual cycles and more painful periods in women. It can also decrease libido (sexual desire) in both men and women.

Common Signs and Symptoms of Stress

Our bodies are designed to handle small doses of short-term stress, but we aren't equipped to handle long-term, chronic stress without harmful consequences. In addition to the physiological repercussions outlined above, stress can affect general physical health and all areas of life, including behavior, emotions, mood, and the ability to think clearly. Symptoms of many pre-existing medical conditions may also worsen during times of stress. There is virtually no part of the body that's immune to it.

Sometimes people become so accustomed to living with stress that they don't know how to identify it and aren't fully aware of its specific effects on them. Here are just a few of the countless warning signs that stress is wreaking havoc on a person's body and mind:

- acid reflux
- chest pain
- confusion
- constipation
- depression
- diarrhea
- difficulty breathing
- excessive sweating
- fatigue
- frequent headaches
- frequent urination
- heartburn
- increased anger and hostility
- jaw clenching
- loss of appetite
- low energy
- muscle spasms
- nausea
- overeating
- poor judgment
- racing thoughts
- sleep changes/insomnia
- stomach pain
- suicidal thoughts
- tremors
- wild mood swings

The Evolution of Stress and Health

Today's stress differs greatly not only from what our evolutionary ancestors faced but also from what our ancestors of just the past century or two experienced. Over the course of human evolution, the stress response has helped the human species survive and deal with environmental challenges by supplying physiological coping mechanisms that impart the energy and quick-thinking skills needed to fight off attackers or escape deadly situations.

Contrarily, contemporary stress mostly originates from the ongoing pressures of daily living as well as fear and worry about what *might* happen in the future, and yet our bodies respond in the same ways as those of our prehistoric predecessors. When the stress response is constantly being engaged, it regularly floods the body with stress hormones and taxes the normal functioning of the body's systems. Modern stress is often chronic and typically arises from circumstances over which we have little control. Our response to it has become ingrained and habituated, but in most instances it provides no benefit to us. Instead, this ceaseless, acculturated stress has been implicated as a primary contributor to an impressive array of "twenty-first-century diseases," including anxiety, cancer, depression, high blood pressure, gastrointestinal dysfunction, neurological disorders (such as Parkinson's disease), immune system disorders (including multiple sclerosis and rheumatoid arthritis), stroke, and many others. In fact, it's difficult to think of any condition that stress doesn't instigate or aggravate to one degree or another, and a growing number of researchers have come to believe that stress could actually be the genesis of all modern diseases.

The Essential Adrenals

Meet the Adrenal Glands

The adrenal glands, also known as suprarenal glands, are small, walnut-sized, triangular-shaped glands located on top of both kidneys. Their name correlates to their location in the body: *ad*, meaning "near" or "at," and *renes*, meaning "kidneys." Surprisingly, the glands aren't symmetrical. The right adrenal gland is triangular, and the left adrenal gland is shaped more like a half-moon. They each have a yellowish hue and are about two and a half inches in length and one inch wide.

The adrenals have three distinct components: the adipose capsule, the cortex, and the medulla. The capsule is a protective layer of fat that surrounds each gland. Although this layer isn't technically part of the glands themselves, its purpose is to enclose and protect each of the adrenals. The adrenal cortex is the outer region and comprises about 80 percent of the volume of the gland. It fully surrounds the adrenal medulla, which sits in the center. The adrenal cortex is composed of three individual zones that perform slightly different functions. The innermost region of the adrenal gland is the medulla. It's surrounded by the adrenal cortex and comprises only 20 percent of the gland's volume. Unlike the cortex, the medulla does not have separate zones.

The role of the adrenal glands is to release certain hormones, many of which have to do with how the body responds to stress, directly into the bloodstream. Although there is some interaction between the adrenal cortex and the adrenal medulla, each performs distinct and separate functions and secretes specific hormones. One of the primary differences between them is that the hormones released by the adrenal cortex are essential to life and those secreted by the adrenal medulla are not.

"Adrenal Fatigue" Deconstructed

The Adrenal Fatigue Enigma

"Adrenal fatigue" is a constellation of diverse medical signs and symptoms, known as a syndrome, that is believed to result when the adrenal glands, along with the hypothalamus and pituitary gland, are functioning below their optimal levels as a result of chronic physical or emotional stress or the outcome of a lifetime of stress that takes a toll as we age. Although the concept of adrenal fatigue has become popularized among alternative health practitioners, the term and condition are not recognized by any endocrinology society or medical group.

Theoretically, adrenal fatigue occurs when hormone levels drop, but unlike Addison's disease, they don't drop low enough for current medical tests to detect an insufficiency. Consequently, laboratory results appear normal.

The adrenal glands perform a variety of vital functions that are essential to life. These include, among others, controlling the body's response to stress, regulating blood pressure and heart rate, supporting the immune system, balancing the levels of salt and water in the body, and aiding the metabolism of carbohydrates, proteins, and fats. Proponents of adrenal fatigue syndrome believe that as we age or when we experience prolonged periods of stress, the adrenal glands begin to weaken, just like other parts of the body over time. They contend that the adrenals may eventually become incapable of responding adequately when they're needed.

Clinical adrenal dysfunction isn't acknowledged by conventional medicine until the adrenal glands virtually stop working and the condition becomes life-threatening (Addison's disease). With purported adrenal fatigue, however, speculation is that the adrenals and related organs are still doing their jobs, but their performance levels are subpar. Although the results of standard medical tests may show hormone levels in the "normal" range, the patient is suffering nonetheless.

The HPA Axis

Although the term "stress" rightfully carries many negative connotations, it describes an important neurobehavioral and physiological response that is intrinsic to life. When confronted with an environmental stressor, the body quickly orchestrates changes in brain activity that are followed shortly thereafter by the secretion of what are called stress mediators. These circulating chemical messages then act in the brain and on peripheral tissues to modify physiological processes and behavioral effects. The primary pathway that regulates our stress response is known as the hypothalamic-pituitary-adrenal (HPA) axis. The stress response coordinated by the HPA axis is a well-choreographed, multisystem response involving behavioral, physiological, and metabolic actions, with tightly regulated components that must be activated at the right time and in the right context.

Normal functioning of the HPA axis ensures that the body responds appropriately to altered environmental demands, equipping it with an essential system to promote survival. Stress activates the HPA axis, initiating a cascade of neuroendocrine signals that trigger the release of hormones and neurotransmitters, such as cortisol, epinephrine (adrenaline), and norepinephrine (noradrenaline). Persistent activation of the stress-response system can, over time, undermine the ability of cells, tissues, and organ systems to rapidly respond to changes in physiological need and can compromise the long-term capability of the body to respond to these changes.

HPA Axis Dysfunction

Allostasis, which literally means "maintaining stability," is the process by which a state of internal, physiological balance (homeostasis) is maintained in response to actual or perceived environmental or psychological stressors.

The body responds to stress with self-regulating, allostatic processes aimed at returning critical systems to a set point within a narrow range of operation that ensures the body's survival. These self-regulating processes include multiple behavioral and physiological components.

Over the past several decades, increasing evidence supports the hypothesis that disruption of the HPA axis can lead to a dysregulated stress response, exacting a physiological toll commonly referred to as allostatic load. The concept of allostatic load was proposed to refer to the wear and tear the body experiences due to repeated cycles of allostasis, as well as to the inefficient turning on and shutting off of these responses. Researchers have acknowledged that a high allostatic load can contribute to increased health vulnerabilities and inappropriate responses to stressors that might underlie abnormal coping strategies and many neuropsychiatric disorders, such as anxiety and depression.

The stress response is an essential brain–body reaction that protects homeostasis and ensures survival in the face of threatening environmental stimuli. This coordinated response that follows a stressful situation allows mediators of allostasis to mobilize, letting the body adapt to a temporary environmental shift. As such, healthy allostatic responses are protective and a sign of resilience. However, if allostatic mediators are overactive, improperly regulated, poorly terminated, or engaged inappropriately, the allostatic burden can increase. Eventually this results in allostatic overload, which, rather than protecting the body, leads to a stream of failures in multiple physiological systems. Consequently, the systems that usually impart resilience result instead in increased vulnerability.

Given the central role of the HPA axis stress response in allostatic processes, it's not surprising that disruptions in the biological reaction to stress can lead to changes in nerve impulse function, behavior, and immune function and can also contribute to negative physical and mental health outcomes. In fact, disruption of normal HPA function is a hallmark of a varied set of physical and neuropsychiatric diseases, including anxiety disorders, depression, post-traumatic stress disorder (PTSD), and metabolic dysfunction. These conditions affect millions of people worldwide, saddling them with significant economic and personal burdens. Whether these changes in HPA activity are a cause or consequence of such disease states is currently unclear, but it's reasonable to speculate that disrupting the normal self-regulating responses to environmental stress will predispose individuals to detrimental health outcomes.

To protect against prolonged hormonal activity, the HPA axis is carefully modulated through negative feedback loops designed to maintain predetermined hormone levels (set points) and homeostasis. These delicately balanced negative feedback mechanisms keep the secretion of ACTH and cortisol within a comparatively narrow range. This function is exceedingly important, because too much or too little exposure to cortisol can have adverse consequences to overall health and result in serious harm to the body.

When a person experiences prolonged chronic stress, the normal release of hormones via the HPA axis is accelerated. In time, the overproduction of these hormones desensitizes the affiliated glands of the HPA axis, and they no longer recognize the signals to stop producing hormones. In other words, the negative feedback loop ceases to work as it should, and HPA axis dysfunction becomes habituated.

Although proponents of "adrenal fatigue" focus on the adrenal glands being fatigued as a result of chronic stress, that is only one possible piece of the puzzle. More likely, if such a syndrome exists, it is the potential dysfunction of the entire HPA axis and its feedback loops that are causing symptoms, not merely a dysfunction in the adrenal glands.

Adrenal Fatigue and the Disease Continuum

Supporters of the concept of adrenal fatigue believe the syndrome could affect millions of people worldwide. However, adrenal fatigue isn't currently an accepted medical diagnosis. It's both interesting and somewhat alarming that such a potentially widespread dysfunction has been castigated by brilliant contemporary physicians around the globe and yet has generated so much interest among the public. Why is there such a wide-scale disconnect?

The basis for conventional medicine rejecting or questioning the existence of adrenal fatigue is multilayered:

1. Is there evidence that chronic, acute, or prolonged stress can lead to an imbalance or suboptimal levels of adrenal hormones?
2. If so, can that reduced hormonal output be quantified?
3. If a quantifiable imbalance exists, can it be proven to be the cause of the reported symptoms?

Neuroscientific research has demonstrated that stress, whether physical or emotional, is a powerful trigger for the release of adrenal hormones, such as adrenaline and cortisol. For example, during times of acute stress, adrenaline levels rapidly rise, and during times of rest, they gradually drop. Although we know that hormone levels are affected by stress, the degree to which these levels rise and fall varies greatly from person to person, and in some people these fluctuations may be barely noticeable. Also, when stress is chronic, these types of acute hormonal shifts don't occur. It's not surprising that laboratory measurements of "stress hormones" differ widely depending on the individual, the circumstances, and the type and level of stress experienced. So while it's clear that stress contributes to hormone imbalance in various ways, subclinical levels can't yet be accurately quantified and therefore don't meet the threshold for what conventional medicine considers scientific evidence.

Do subclinical hormone imbalances lead to clinical symptoms of fatigue? Because of the enormous variances among individuals, it's possible that some people could have clinically abnormal adrenaline output yet not feel fatigued, while other people may feel exhausted but their adrenaline levels are in the normal range. At this time there are no quantitative tests that can accurately show a conclusive connection between particular levels of any single adrenal hormone and symptoms of fatigue.

On the one hand, because current laboratory tests don't have the capacity to measure subclinical states, these tests may not realistically be useful for diagnosing adrenal fatigue. On the other hand, it's possible the current tests have value, but the reference ranges need to be readjusted or the thresholds lowered to accurately reflect subclinical states.

We know conclusively that many degenerative diseases and common causes of death, including heart disease and cancer, can take several years or even decades to develop before symptoms are clinically detectable. However, our current laboratory tests and clinical detection methods lack the sensitivity to identify the signs of early disease. Although a person may appear outwardly healthy, genetic predisposition or a lifetime of poor nutrition, stress, and exposure to environmental contaminants may be taking an imperceptible toll.

It's not unusual for a person to feel seriously ill yet appear to be symptom-free and have normal laboratory test results. Conventional medicine generally refrains from labeling a person as ill until the threshold for what's considered normal in terms of laboratory value references is crossed. These value references are derived from data based on the general population, and for that reason they don't and can't incorporate or reflect the broad range of individual variances.

So while modern testing methods are tremendously valuable for diagnosing catastrophic illness, they presently are incapable of detecting subclinical progressive disease states, such as borderline adrenal dysfunction and borderline hormonal, metabolic, or electrolyte imbalances. The current medical framework defines "normal" as the absence of any detectable illness exhibited by laboratory test results that fall within a statistical range based on mathematical averages. Therefore, if lab results don't reflect the minimum standardized levels for suboptimal function, the patient will be deemed healthy, despite contrary symptomatology. In other words, a person is considered either healthy or sick—there's no continuum or in-between stage.

If there's no demonstrable pathology to define a disease state, then according to conventional medicine, disease is nonexistent. But because the threshold for what is considered normal or abnormal is based on averages, not individuals, using laboratory testing as the sole definitive diagnostic tool is inherently flawed. Many people who have normal test results may be ill, but they're told that nothing is wrong with them and they're ushered out of the doctor's office and sent home. However, by the time laboratory tests detect a problem, the illness may have advanced too far to be treatable. Both scenarios do patients a disservice and cause needless suffering. Every untreated chronic or serious illness, from cancer to diabetes to hypertension, progresses from normal to severe over time, so it's only common sense that mild dysfunction of the adrenal glands or HPA axis exists, regardless of what it's called.

Conventional medicine has dismissed claims of adrenal fatigue in much the same way it once rejected claims of other syndromes, such as chronic fatigue syndrome (CFS), fibromyalgia, premenstrual syndrome (PMS), Raynaud's syndrome, and irritable bowel syndrome (IBS), for which no standardized medical tests currently exist. Although mainstream physicians don't refute the symptoms of "adrenal fatigue" as reported by sufferers, they believe the root cause of these symptoms lies outside the adrenal glands and is more likely attributable to depression, CFS, or fibromyalgia than adrenal issues. What's fascinating is that not all that long ago, conventional medicine considered these very same diagnoses baseless.

Contrarily, practitioners of natural and alternative medicine, including naturopathic physicians and practitioners of functional, integrative, and traditional Chinese medicine, acknowledge the existence of adrenal fatigue syndrome and offer treatments for it. However, conventional physicians argue that accepting a medically unrecognized diagnosis from an "unqualified" health-care practitioner and using unproven remedies could make a patient feel worse because the true underlying cause of the symptoms remains undiagnosed and untreated. Bearing in mind the turnabout of the medical establishment with regard to other syndromes it once considered invalid but has now come to recognize, study, and even treat, would it be prudent to similarly embrace the possibility that adrenal fatigue syndrome is real?

Perhaps. But that approach is also a common and clever strategy for creating lucrative "fake" diseases, because knowing where to draw the line between what is healthy and unhealthy is a genuine medical quandary. It's easy for unscrupulous practitioners to take a true medical condition (such as adrenal insufficiency) and claim that a milder version of it (i.e., adrenal fatigue) also constitutes a real disease. For example, doctors have long debated where to draw the line between normal blood pressure and hypertension. The line keeps moving, and that's a legitimate medical controversy. Probably the best way to resolve these concerns is to conduct clinical studies to determine who benefits from treatment: the patient or the practitioner.

Symptoms of "Adrenal Fatigue"

The condition referred to as adrenal fatigue syndrome (AFS) is associated with myriad signs and symptoms, and each of these symptoms conceivably can be connected to a possible deficiency in one or more of the hormones produced by the HPA axis. Currently there is no definitive laboratory test to confirm or disconfirm a diagnosis of AFS, but if a person is suffering from a high number of these symptoms, champions of AFS would say it points to "adrenal fatigue" as the likely cause.

Ideally cortisol levels fluctuate according to circadian cycles, peaking in the morning and decreasing incrementally to a low at bedtime, only to rise again overnight. Among the hallmarks of purported adrenal fatigue are cortisol levels that are too high at night and not high enough in the morning. Alternative health practitioners contend that one reason standard blood tests are unable to detect these irregularities is because the tests are performed at whatever time is convenient for the doctor or laboratory, whereas a more effective diagnostic approach would be to test hormone levels at various times of the day, as doing so is far more likely to reveal an abnormal pattern of cortisol or dehydroepiandrosterone (DHEA) secretion.

Unlike adrenal insufficiency and adrenal crisis, adrenal fatigue syndrome, if it exists, isn't life-threatening. However, because the causes of these conditions and the presumed cause of "adrenal fatigue" are similar (reduced or erratic secretion of adrenal hormones), it's not surprising that many symptoms of alleged adrenal fatigue parallel those of adrenal insufficiency. The most common symptoms associated with AFS include the following:

- alternating diarrhea and constipation
- anxiety
- body aches
- changes in appetite
- cravings for salty foods
- decreased ability to handle stress
- depression
- difficulty getting out of bed in the morning
- difficulty recovering from infections
- digestive problems
- disinterest in sex
- dry skin
- fatigue that's unrelieved by sleep
- heart palpitations
- high incidence of flu and other respiratory illnesses
- higher energy levels in the evenings
- hypoglycemia (low blood sugar)
- insomnia despite being tired
- joint pain
- lethargy
- low body temperature
- memory problems
- mood disorders
- multiple food and/or environmental allergies
- muscle weakness
- overuse of stimulants, such as caffeine and sugar
- panic attacks
- premature menopause
- rage attacks
- recurrent infections
- sleep disturbances
- thinning of the skin
- trouble thinking clearly (brain fog)
- unexplained hair loss
- unexplained pain in upper back or neck
- worsening PMS symptoms

Potential Causes of "Adrenal Fatigue"

The purpose of the adrenal glands is to adapt the body to stressors. A natural cycle of stress, adaptation, and recovery allows the body to acclimate to environmental changes and stimuli and grow stronger through the process. However, when stressors override our ability to adapt effectively, or if the stress response is chronic, the body's vital reserves become depleted, impeding the body's ability to heal itself.

Excessive stress can arise from a variety of diverse sources. Contributing to our physical burden of stress are addictions (drug or alcohol), chemical exposure, chronic illness, disease, injury, overuse of drugs (pharmaceuticals, illicit drugs, over-the-counter medications), pollution, recurrent infections, and surgery. But stress may also be due to psychological or emotional factors, including the daily demands of modern life, mental illness or mental health problems, work difficulties, worry, and a host of chronic health and lifestyle factors. Among these are chronic infections, environmental toxins, nutritional deficiencies, excessive exercise, and stimulants in the form of drugs (pharmaceuticals, over-the-counter, and recreational) or socially acceptable stimulants that people consume on a regular basis, such as alcohol, caffeine, chocolate, and sugar.

Diagnosing "Adrenal Fatigue"

"Adrenal fatigue" could be described as a cluster of symptoms that disrupt a person's regular ability to function. As yet, it can't be accounted for by a single pathognomonic marker or a medically acknowledged condition because the symptoms don't have a clear indication of etiology. Consequently there isn't any one test that can confirm a diagnosis. Instead, so-called adrenal fatigue, like many other syndromes, is typically identified through a process of exclusion. This means that serious and medically recognized conditions must be ruled out as a cause for these diverse symptoms. Because the HPA axis can be affected by several chronic and/or metabolic disorders, other primary conditions must be excluded before intrinsic disorders of the HPA axis can be deemed responsible. When patients complain of symptoms, practitioners of conventional and complementary medicine typically order a range of tests, some of which may be conducted multiple times, and record every symptom reported. This requires not only experience but also a thorough knowledge of the various body systems. In addition, several office visits may be necessary before an accurate diagnosis can be made, so the process typically requires a fair amount of patience.

Screening for adrenal dysfunction may include standard hormone tests that measure cortisol and various thyroid hormone levels. To correctly make a diagnosis, a combination of lab testing, physical examinations with patient feedback, and questionnaires have been shown to be useful.

Additional Tests

Several additional tests may be recommended by alternative health practitioners for patients reporting symptoms associated with presumed adrenal fatigue syndrome. However, most of these tests are based on little more than wishful thinking and speculation, not science. While physically harmless, be aware that they could be misleading, offer false hope or unnecessary fear, and potentially delay treatment for more serious, underlying conditions.

Hair, tissue, mineral analysis (HTMA). Hair analysis is a test in which a sample of a person's hair (typically from the back of the neck) is sent to a laboratory for measurement of its mineral content. This test is often used by chiropractors, "nutritional consultants," and alternative health-care practitioners as a basis for prescribing supplements.

Iris contraction test (pupillary reflex). Normally the pupil of the eye will hold a steady contraction when it's exposed to light, which means that it will get smaller and will usually stay that way. This self-test measures the contraction of the iris in response to repeated exposure to dark light. Theoretically, in people with weakened adrenal function, the iris will be unable to maintain its contraction for very long. Alternatively, the pupil may not contract at all, or it might contract and then quickly dilate, or it might move from contraction to dilation.

To conduct the test, sit in front of a mirror in a darkened room. Take a weak flashlight or penlight and shine it across one eye from the side of your head, keeping the flashlight about six inches from your face (don't shine the light directly in the eye). According to the purported theory, if a person is in a hypoadrenal state (that is, their adrenal glands are underactive), the pupil will not be able to hold the contraction for longer than two minutes and will begin to dilate despite the light shining on it. In people with healthy adrenals, according to the theory, the contraction should last much longer.

Lower-than-normal body temperature. The normal human body temperature is 98 degrees F, but for some people the normal baseline temperature is lower. In addition, some people may notice a minor decrease in their normal body temperature as they age. What's "normal" may vary somewhat depending on how, where, and when the temperature is taken. There are a number of possible causes for a lower-than-normal body temperature other than adrenal abnormalities, including acute infection, kidney disease, and hypothyroidism (which can slow the body's metabolism). If a person's body temperature has dropped to an unusually low level, medical help should be sought immediately.

Postural low blood pressure (Ragland's sign). When people who are in good health stand up, there is an almost immediate rise in blood pressure. Hypothetically, people who suffer from adrenal fatigue will see no change in their blood pressure upon standing or may even see a slight drop. Broadly speaking, the theory goes that the larger the drop in blood pressure, the more severe the case of adrenal fatigue.

Rogoff's sign. More of a symptom than a test, this refers to pain in the midback region, where the ribs are located, that feels similar to a kidney infection, pulled muscle, or strained ligament.

Salivary hormone testing. Most salivary hormone tests are available online and can be obtained without a prescription. These tests measure the amount of free cortisol and dehydroepiandrosterone (DHEA), among other hormones, found in the saliva. Salivary hormone levels may vary according to the time of day the saliva is collected, the person's diet, or the person's level of hydration. Thus the timing of the saliva collection may affect the results, and the salivary flow rate can affect the concentration of certain hormones. Different laboratories may require different testing methods, such as obtaining several samples over a couple of weeks at specific times of the day. The results of these tests are often used to determine a supposed need for prescriptions for DHEA, vitamins, minerals, herbs, and other supplements. Meta-analysis of the scientific literature shows that researchers question the value and validity of patients supplementing with DHEA to improve health outcomes.

White line test. This test is self-administered. Uncover the abdomen or the inner forearm for fifteen minutes so the skin can be seen in good light. Use the dull end of a ballpoint pen or a chopstick and lightly stroke the skin of the abdomen, making a mark about six inches in length; be sure not to scratch or break the skin's surface. Within a few seconds a line will appear. Theoretically, people with normal adrenal function will show an initial white line that will turn red in fifteen to twenty seconds, but if adrenal fatigue is present, the line will stay white for about two minutes and widen, but no red line will appear.

Science versus Subjectivity

Is adrenal fatigue syndrome real? The answer isn't simple, and it probably depends on who you ask. But as yet, there is no substantiation in the scientific literature to prove its existence. The reported symptoms of adrenal fatigue are, for the most part, broad and unspecific. While the symptoms themselves are no doubt real, they easily overlap with other known medical issues. But the primary concern is that the reported symptoms are not objective or measurable by current methodologies. In other words, there are no valid tests or reliable symptom scores to assess how mild or severe a case may be. Consequently, without any means to accurately measure the severity of the "syndrome," there is no way to accurately measure the effectiveness of any treatment that may be prescribed for it.

Theories on adrenal impairment as the source of fatigue are alluring because they offer up a treatable condition; it's simply human nature to want to make sense of patterns and clusters of symptoms and attempt to label them. But it's critical to determine whether there's a true correlation between adrenal status and fatigue states or fatigue-related diseases and to examine the results of any peer-reviewed studies correlating cortisol and fatigue.

Obviously there is a divide between the scientific community, alternative practitioners, and the general public regarding this supposed condition. There currently are no approved, reliable, or consistent methods to clinically screen for alleged adrenal fatigue. Although validated surveys have been used in studies that investigated fatigue states, they weren't correlated with proper cortisol assessment methods.

Functional tests (those that identify, interpret, and quantify systems of dysfunction) are the only methods endorsed by endocrinology societies to assess adrenal cortisol production. But there has been conflicting data using these tests when trying to differentiate exhausted, fatigued individuals from healthy patients, such as an unexpected increase (rather than decrease) in cortisol levels in fatigued subjects in selected studies, rendering these methods unusable in terms of differentiating fatigued from non-fatigued individuals.

An important consideration is whether cortisol markers can be used to assess cortisol impairment. Major tests used to identify underlying causes of the fatigue state have been unable to demonstrate significant differences or causality in heterogeneous groups of subjects, since the etiology and pathogenesis of fatigue status could be the consequence of other disorders, such as sleep disturbances.

Adrenal size could be considered another marker of adrenal activity, as the enlargement of the adrenal glands could be the result of ACTH over-stimulation by the pituitary glands, and an atrophic (diminished) gland may reflect adrenal insufficiency at any level of the HPA axis. However, there has been little to no research to date in which adrenal size has been checked in fatigued or exhausted patients. Finally, none of these as yet has been shown to be an accurate marker of fatigue, and studies haven't correlated them with HPA axis dysfunction as an etiology of fatigue.

An extensive meta-analysis conducted by endocrinologists to examine a possible correlation between the HPA axis, "adrenal fatigue," and other conditions associated with fatigue, exhaustion, or burnout has been unable to demonstrate the existence of adrenal fatigue. In order for adrenal fatigue to be substantiated, further investigation is required by the groups that claim it exists, and those studies must employ the most appropriate scientific methods to assess the correlation between stress, fatigue, and the HPA axis.

Fact versus Fake

How can you tell when a theorized syndrome is an actual medical condition? A true medical condition is a distinct clinical entity with something specific about one or more of the symptoms or a combination of symptoms. A collection of common, nonspecific symptoms doesn't constitute a clinical entity. A specific biomarker, such as a laboratory test or study that confirms an abnormal result that will respond to specific treatment, also provides validity.

"Fake" diseases are fabricated without any objective, empirical evidence to confirm their existence. They emerge from vague symptoms that can't be attributed to any particular medical condition, giving an alternative health provider broad leeway in providing a fictitious diagnosis and treatment plan, even if the condition is completely unsubstantiated or possibly made up. Because the diagnosis guides the treatment plan (or ought to), it's essential to get the diagnosis right. That means running proven tests to rule out serious illness rather than practitioners jumping to a preferred diagnosis and treatment, which is frequently the case when it comes to adrenal fatigue.

Fraudulent syndromes are often confirmed by laboratory tests that are misused or misinterpreted to provide bogus legitimacy for a questionable diagnosis. For instance, these tests may be designed to produce false positives, while medically valid tests with verifiable diagnostic criteria may be dismissed as inappropriate or ill-advised. In the case of adrenal fatigue, highly variable tests, such as the saliva test for cortisol, might be given many times until the practitioner obtains the desired result. This type of test is ideal for generating false positives, so it's popular among advocates of adrenal fatigue.

At this time the only "evidence" proffered by adrenal fatigue specialists is anecdotal. Typically when the patient makes a few healthy lifestyle changes in conjunction with either real or dubious treatment, and positive outcomes result, the dubious treatment receives credit. The story might unfold along these lines: "I was tired and depressed, but my regular physician found nothing wrong with me. Then I went to Dr. X and was diagnosed with adrenal fatigue. Following Dr. X's advice, I changed my diet, began exercising, and worked on controlling my stress. I also took Dr. X's magic tonic every day. I was shocked how well the magic tonic worked! One year later, I'm feeling great!"

Real diseases and syndromes, along with treatments for them, are supported by a body of scientific literature. But dubious practitioners with self-invented (and often self-serving) diagnoses and conspiracy theories about how dreadful conventional medicine is and how fabulous their alternative treatments are don't have a scientific foundation. That's not to say that mainstream medicine doesn't have its faults and failings. Inarguably, it's not perfect. However, that's not a good reason to accept unsubstantiated, misleading, and potentially harmful claims.

But what about other legitimate medical diagnoses that aren't yet detectable by tests? Diagnoses such as dementia, depression, irritable bowel syndrome, and Parkinson's disease are often determined and treated based on symptoms, not the results of lab tests. While that's certainly true, many fabricated syndromes are used to exploit susceptible people who are merely dealing with common symptoms that are the fallout of contemporary life. Some of these individuals may actually have a real underlying disease, but they may get distracted from investigating an authentic diagnosis when a fake one is readily offered up instead. For many people, lifestyle adjustments are all they need to improve their health, and that may be the best place for them to focus their efforts, rather than on magic supplements and elixirs to treat syndromes that are not yet confirmed and may very well be fictitious.

Next Steps

For people who constantly feel unwell, it's incredibly frustrating to have a doctor be unable or unwilling to discover their true problem. That's completely understandable, because the symptoms a patient is experiencing are real. Indeed, that's why people often turn to alternative practitioners and why alternative practitioners often label their patients' cluster of symptoms as adrenal fatigue. A tangible diagnosis gives patients hope that whatever they're dealing with can be cured. It also opens the door for these same health-care providers to sell untested, unproven supplements to optimistic, impressionable, or desperate patients and profit from them. However, with no scientific evidence to substantiate the concept of adrenal fatigue and no reliable method of detecting, measuring, or resolving it, it's impossible to make such a diagnosis (at least not one that's valid) or recommend therapies or prescribe appropriate remedies. At what point do any potential benefits of unwarranted or spurious treatments outweigh the risks and expense?

Nevertheless, a diagnosis of adrenal fatigue could have some unexpected advantages. When people have a specific reason to take action and adjust their lifestyles, improve their diets, and reduce their stressors, they're often motivated to do so. That's one reason so many individuals with supposed adrenal fatigue who are given a treatment plan that includes positive lifestyle changes end up experiencing improvement and feeling better.

But what if the real issue is deeper and more complex than simply poor diet and high stress? Accepting adrenal fatigue as the primary reason for symptoms can be dangerous because it will prolong the time required to discover what's actually the root cause. Conventional doctors urge patients to not waste precious time accepting an unproven diagnosis of adrenal fatigue. Instead, they encourage anyone who is feeling exhausted, weak, chronically ill, hopeless, or sad to obtain a medically accepted diagnosis so the true source of those symptoms—such as adrenal insufficiency, depression, obstructive sleep apnea, or other health problems—can be properly explored and treated.

Practitioners who support the notion of adrenal fatigue may advise their patients to make important lifestyle adjustments, such as giving up alcohol, drugs, caffeine, and smoking. They may also suggest starting an exercise program, eating healthier foods, and following a regular daily routine for sleeping and waking. These types of lifestyle changes almost always help people feel better, no matter what medical diagnosis they've been given. But these practitioners may also encourage their patients to undergo various tests or buy special supplements and vitamins that the practitioners themselves have formulated or that they claim have been developed specifically for adrenal health and support. People who don't feel well are yearning for answers and solutions, which makes them easy prey for naïve, inexperienced, or shady practitioners who may be eager to sell these unproven, expensive, and even potentially harmful tests, supplements, and treatments. Although some ordinary vitamins and minerals might be health supportive for certain conditions, taking supplements sold as a treatment for adrenal fatigue could be risky. Nutrition supplements should be used to address known deficiencies linked with particular conditions, but only a handful of scientific studies even mention the term "adrenal fatigue," let alone have tested for associated nutrient deficiencies.

The US Food and Drug Administration (the governmental arm that oversees most food and medical products in the United States) doesn't regulate nutritional supplements and vitamins. This means there's no guarantee that what's on the label of a supplement is actually what's inside the bottle. Laboratory testing has shown that some supplements have very few, if any, active ingredients, and in others the dose of a particular ingredient has been found to be too high. This is often the case if the supplements are purchased from a compounding pharmacy, where they are made directly by the pharmacist. There are also many hormone supplements available that promise to treat adrenal fatigue, but taking adrenal hormone supplements when they aren't needed can do far more harm than good and may instigate adrenal crisis, a potentially life-threatening condition.

Getting an accurate and legitimate diagnosis is crucial for any person who feels ill or whose well-being has been compromised. Even though it's disheartening for patients to have symptoms that defy diagnosis, heeding advice from unqualified practitioners can be ineffective at best and dangerous or even deadly at worst. Beware of any website or practitioner that diagnoses an illness and also sells the cure.

Whether or not adrenal fatigue exists, taking measures to improve your diet, overhaul harmful habits, and better manage life's stressors are the safest and surest keys to regaining your health. There are proven methods to do each of these that will benefit almost anyone who has received a diagnosis of "adrenal fatigue," or even people who have received a clean bill of health from their doctors despite experiencing many of the symptoms commonly associated with alleged adrenal fatigue. Although changing ingrained patterns and lifelong habits requires more effort, diligence, and discipline than popping a pill or taking a potion, the upshot is a stronger body and a healthier mind so you can endure and overcome the challenges life throws at you.

Stress Management

Stress is at the core of presumed adrenal fatigue, because it's the body's response to stress that ignites the flow of "stress hormones" from the HPA axis, and it's the resolution of stress that signals negative feedback loops to halt that hormonal release. Consequently, knowing how to manage stress levels is a crucial first step in getting a handle on any potential health issues associated with possible stress-related hormone imbalances, "adrenal fatigue," or HPA axis dysfunction.

Contemporary life is teeming with stress, and it may seem as though there's little we can do to minimize it. Bills pile up, we need more hours in the day, and work and home responsibilities are relentless. But you actually have more control over stress than you may realize. At the heart of stress management is learning how to effectively master bad habits, handle obsessive thoughts and emotions, and take charge of problems. Regardless of how stressful life seems, there are steps we all can take to relieve the pressure, regain control, restore our health, and reclaim our lives.

While there's currently no scientific evidence that stress depletes our adrenal hormones or causes damage to the adrenal glands or the HPA axis, there's no question that living with high levels of stress can take a toll on a person's health and put emotional equilibrium and overall well-being in jeopardy. Chronic stress clouds thinking, impedes the ability to function, and hinders the ability to enjoy life.

However, effective stress management can break the hold stress has on our lives so we can be happier, healthier, and more productive. The ultimate goal is balance: achieving the resilience to stand up to pressure and meet life's challenges head on while ensuring sufficient time and energy for work, relationships, relaxation, and fun. But stress management is not a one-size-fits-all approach. It's important to explore and experiment to discover what works best for you and your individual needs, preferences, and circumstances.

First, try to identify your stressors. While major life events (such as buying a house or going through a divorce) tend to be obvious, the sources of chronic stress are usually far more subtle and complicated. Pay attention to how you react to difficult situations and how your stress levels increase because of negative self-talk and harmful beliefs and attitudes. In many ways we're often responsible for contributing to ongoing stress and are our own worst enemies. But the upside of this is that we can be equally instrumental in changing our response to stressful situations. If we have a hand in worsening our stress levels, then it's also within our power to improve them.

Second, adopt healthy coping strategies. Take a look at how you respond to the stressors in your life so you can determine whether your approaches are healthy and helpful or obstructive and damaging. If your current methods of dealing with stress aren't supporting your emotional and physical health, it's crucial that you find other ways of coping that are more constructive. You can experiment with a wide range of approaches to discover which ones fit your needs and help you calm down and feel in control. The suggestions that follow will give you a good start in finding options to explore.

Change Your Response to Stressful Situations

Although you can't control your autonomic nervous system's response to stress, there are some stressors in life you can anticipate and prepare for. When these arise, you can either avoid or change the situation or alter your response to it by following these tips:

Reclaim your power. While it's never wise to evade responsibilities or dodge a situation that needs to be addressed, when circumstances are unworkable or you've reached the breaking point, it's essential to take back your power or walk away. Discover how much you can handle and what your limits are. Differentiate between what you think you *should* do and what you truly *need* to do. Learn how to say no and stand your ground.

Limit stressful experiences. If certain people or situations make you feel anxious, uncomfortable, or on edge, you don't have to be involved with them. Minimize the time you spend with toxic individuals, especially your time alone with them, or terminate your relationship if that's the only realistic solution. Avoid stress-producing experiences whenever possible. If you know something will upset you (such as reading about current events or watching scary movies), find more calming, soothing options.

Communicate. Discussing what you're feeling or going through can be a remarkable stress reliever, even if there isn't anything you can do to change the situation. If you don't have someone you trust to talk with, make an appointment with a therapist or write down your thoughts in a journal. Bottling up emotions is unhealthy, and it also feeds feelings of anger and bitterness that could lead to hostility, violent behavior, or depression. If someone or something is annoying you, speak up rather than holding in your feelings and letting resentment build. Learn how to communicate your concerns in a manner that's honest, respectful, and constructive.

Laugh about it. A sense of humor in trying times releases tension, decreases levels of stress hormones, lowers blood pressure, reduces anxiety, and helps maintain perspective. Sometimes just laughing about the absurdity of the situation is all that's needed to get you through it.

Accept what you can't change. Many aspects of life are beyond our control, including what other people say and do. Often the best way to cope with adversity is to simply accept things as they are. While there's no doubt that acceptance may be difficult, in the long run it's easier than railing against an immutable situation. Rather than letting your circumstances stress you out, focus on what you *can* control, such as how you respond to difficult people, problems, and challenges.

Move Your Body

Although exercise may be one of the last things you feel like doing when you're stressed out, moderate physical activity is among the top best stress relievers. In addition to being a valuable distraction from daily worries, exercise releases endorphins, the "feel good" hormones that enhance mood and boost energy. Exercise also reduces anxiety and depression and enhances sleep.

You don't have to become an athlete or spend hours at the gym to reap the benefits of movement. While exercising for thirty minutes five to seven days a week will provide the greatest benefits, you can build up your fitness level gradually or distribute your activity in small increments throughout the day, such as in two fifteen-minute sessions or three ten-minute sessions. Even a single ten-minute walk would be beneficial. The first step, though, is to just get started.

Making exercise a habit takes more than just knowing how and why to do it; it requires the right mind-set and an intelligent approach. Whatever your age or fitness level, there are measures you can take to make exercise less intimidating and more fun and instinctive. A little exercise is better than none at all. In fact, adding just small amounts of physical activity to your daily routine can have an enormous positive effect on your emotional well-being. Start slowly and be gentle with yourself. Try not to be discouraged by what you can't do; focus on consistency instead. You'll be amazed at how quickly you'll see improvements in your mood and energy levels.

Exercise can be used as a form of "meditation in action." Zeroing in on how your body feels as you move and noticing the rhythm of your breath and the flexing of your muscles will not only improve your physical conditioning but will also divert your attention away from negative thoughts and worries, further helping to ease stress and anxiety.

If you're not the type of person who likes to follow a structured exercise program, try thinking about physical activity as a lifestyle choice rather than as a task that must be crossed off your to-do list. Examine your daily routine and look for ways to slip in a bit of extra movement. Even small activities will add up over the course of the day. Housework, gardening, and yard work can be considered exercise too, especially if they're done at a lively pace.

Additional Stress-Relief Approaches

Although stress management can't cure physical illness, it can play a vital role in medical treatments. Specific stress-reduction strategies tend to target specific medical conditions, but in general, the quality of life and well-being of almost anyone will improve when stress is reduced. Bear in mind that what works for one person may not necessarily work for someone else or for you. Also note that some stress-reduction approaches may not be medically approved or have scientific validity, even though many people claim they work for them. Be aware that no single method is always successful; usually a combination of approaches is what turns out to be the most effective.

A number of relaxation exercises can help you to become more aware of muscle tension and other physical sensations of stress. Once you know what the stress response feels like in your body, you can make a conscious effort to practice a relaxation exercise as soon as you start to feel stress symptoms arise. Catching and alleviating stress early on can help prevent it from spiraling out of control.

The more you practice specific stress-reduction techniques, the better you will become at them. Be patient and don't let your efforts to relax turn into yet another stressor. If one stress-relief exercise doesn't seem to work for you, try another. Here are just a few of the many strategies you can explore:

Acupressure

Acupressure is the practice of applying precise pressure, usually with the fingertips, to various tactical points on the body. The objective is to balance a person's energy, or life force, called "qi" in traditional Chinese medicine or "chi" in the West. The pressure points lie along channels of energy in the body known as meridians. Acupressure therapy can be used to relieve pain, reduce muscle tension, improve circulation, and promote deep states of relaxation. Although acupressure is usually provided by massage therapists and other types of bodyworkers, it can also be learned as a self-care technique that individuals can perform on themselves.

Acupuncture

Acupuncture is a holistic treatment mechanism based on traditional Chinese medicine. Acupuncturists believe that illness occurs when something is blocking or imbalancing a person's life energy (known as "qi" or "chi"), and acupuncture is a way to unblock or influence it to flow back into balance. The treatment involves the stimulation of strategic locations on the body by inserting thin, solid metallic needles into the skin. Sometimes heat, pressure, or mild electrical current is used along with the needles. Surprisingly, although needles are used in acupuncture, the treatments are relatively pain-free.

Aromatherapy

Aromatherapy is the therapeutic application of naturally extracted aromatic plant oils, known as essential oils, to promote physical and psychological health. Essential oils are concentrated, volatile extracts taken from the roots, leaves, seeds, or blossoms of plants. Although aromatherapy oils are commonly inhaled using a diffuser, steam bath, or spray to disperse oil droplets into the air, they may also be diluted with a neutral base (such as a lotion or cream) or neutral carrier oil (such as sweet almond oil or olive oil) and applied topically or massaged into the skin. Note that essential oils should not be applied directly to the skin without first being diluted; a few drops of essential oil to an ounce of carrier oil is the usual concentration. Never take essential oils by mouth, as some oils are toxic and ingesting them could be fatal.

Biofeedback

Biofeedback therapy is a noninvasive, drug-free technique that helps patients learn how to control body processes that are normally involuntary, such as blood pressure, heart rate, and muscle tension. Patients are connected to electrical sensors that provide feedback about the body's functions that can help them focus on making subtle changes to achieve the desired results, such as relaxing certain muscles to help reduce pain. Essentially biofeedback gives people the power to use their thoughts to control their bodies to improve various health conditions through teaching relaxation techniques and mental exercises that can alleviate symptoms.

A growing number of biofeedback devices and programs are now being marketed for home use.

Cognitive Behavioral Therapy

Cognitive behavioral therapy is a short-term, goal-oriented approach that basically combines psychotherapy with behavioral therapy. The objective is to modify ingrained behavior or patterns of thinking that contribute to people's problems and, by doing so, change the way they feel.

Deep Breathing

Also called slow abdominal breathing, belly breathing, diaphragmatic breathing, and paced respiration, deep breathing occurs when the air coming through the nose fully fills the lungs and causes the lower part of the belly to rise. Deep breathing is the opposite of "chest breathing," which is the way most people tend to breathe. Chest breathing increases tension and anxiety, whereas deep breathing releases tension and reduces anxiety. That's because shallow chest breathing limits the diaphragm's range of motion, and the lowest part of the lungs doesn't get its full share of oxygenated air. Although shallow breathing may feel "normal," it can make you feel short of breath and anxious. Conversely, deep abdominal breathing encourages a full exchange of oxygen, creating a beneficial trade-off of incoming oxygen for outgoing carbon dioxide. As a result, it lowers or stabilizes blood pressure and slows heart rate.

For a small number of people, breathing exercises can increase anxiety, especially if they aren't practiced correctly. It's important to never force an inhalation or exhalation or try to control your breath. Instead, let your breath come and go naturally. The idea is to simply *observe* your natural breath and slowly count along with it. Trying to create an unnatural breathing pattern will promote stress and tension, which defeats the purpose of the exercise. Just relax, let your breath flow automatically, and watch it in your mind's eye.

Mindfulness-Based Stress Reduction

Mindfulness-Based Stress Reduction (MBSR) is a formal eight-week group program taught by physicians, nurses, psychologists, and social workers, as well as other health professionals. At the core of MBSR is the practice of mindfulness, which involves focusing your attention on one thing in the moment, whether it's each breath you take, each step as you walk, or the sights or sounds around you. The program challenges participants to practice present-moment awareness, deep relaxation, and gentle movement. Through the use of these techniques, participants learn to discover and observe their reactions to life's stressors so they can consciously choose how to respond. With practice, they can then apply these skills to everyday situations.

Progressive Muscle Relaxation

Progressive muscle relaxation (PMR) is a technique that focuses on relaxing each individual muscle group. It's often combined with deep breathing (see page 35) and is simple to learn. Although it's helpful anytime you feel stressed, it's especially useful for promoting sleep, so you might want to do PMR at bedtime. Practicing PMR regularly will make it much more effective and produce a relaxed mental and physical state more rapidly.

To begin, move to a quiet room that's warm but not excessively warm. Make sure you won't be interrupted by other people or the phone, computer, or doorbell. Lie down with your arms and legs uncrossed. Close your eyes and take a deep breath through your nose to a count of 4, hold it for a count of 4, then exhale slowly through your mouth or nose to a count of 8. Repeat three more times. Maintain a slow, deep breathing pattern throughout the entire exercise.

Now concentrate on each part of the body, beginning with the top of your head and progressing downward. Be sure to include the scalp, forehead, ears, eyes, eyelids, mouth, front of the neck, back of the neck, shoulders, upper back, lower back, arms, hands, fingers, chest, belly, buttocks, thighs, calves, feet, toes, and bottoms of the feet. Some people prefer to go in the opposite direction, from the bottom of the feet to the top of the head. Choose which direction you prefer most, and then stick with it.

To further increase your awareness and relaxation, tense each muscle as tightly as possible for a count of 5 to 10, and then release it completely. Experience the muscle as totally relaxed and as heavy as lead. It should feel as though it's sinking deep into the floor or bed. Feel the muscles relax and become loose and limp, and let your whole body and all your cells relax and feel warm and comfortable.

Visualization

Visualization is a technique in which you form mental images to take a visual journey to a calming place or situation that makes you feel happy, relaxed, and peaceful. To relax using visualization, try to incorporate as many senses as possible, including sight, smell, sound, and touch. For instance, if you imagine relaxing in a garden or at a park on a sunny day, think about the smell of the grass and flowers, the sound of a nearby burbling brook, and the warmth of the sun on your face. To begin, sit or lie down in a quiet, comfortable place where you won't be disturbed. Loosen any tight clothing, close your eyes, and concentrate on your breathing as you focus on positive images, experiences, and thoughts.

Self-Hypnosis

One of the principal tenets of hypnosis is inducing a deeply relaxed state, which makes it an ideal tool for both reducing and managing stress. Visit a hypnotherapist or listen to hypnosis CDs. You can also learn some easy and effective self-hypnosis techniques through books or self-help programs to relieve stress. You only need to practice self-hypnosis a few minutes each day or several times a week to help reduce the negative effects of stress on your life and health.

Positive Self-Talk

We all have a set of messages that our minds play over and over again, but too often this internal discourse is negative. One of the most effective ways to overcome these self-sabotaging messages is to "overwrite" them with positive self-talk. Note that this isn't self-deception. Positive self-talk encourages acknowledgment of the many favorable qualities and truths about ourselves that are often obscured or suppressed. By engaging in positive self-talk, you can focus on your strengths, lift yourself up, and remain calm in any given situation.

Massage Therapy

Massage not only feels great, but it has also been shown to be effective in reducing perceived stress and anxiety levels. However, there are several different forms of massage, and although some are relaxing, others may be more stimulating and invigorating. Moderate pressure, as with Swedish massage, tends to lower blood pressure and enhance relaxation, while trigger point therapy and deep tissue massage may actually raise blood pressure. Try different types of massage to find the ones that feel best to you and that make you feel the most relaxed.

Meditation

Meditation has been practiced for thousands of years. Originally intended to deepen human understanding of the esoteric and sacred forces of life, it's primarily used today to produce a deep state of relaxation and a tranquil mind. Meditation involves focused attention (such as on the breath, on an object, or on a prayer or mantra), which helps to eliminate the constant mental chatter that jumbles our thoughts and causes stress. It's simple and inexpensive and doesn't require any special clothing or equipment. It also can be practiced by anyone, regardless of age or health. Meditation can impart a sense of calm, peace, and balance that can benefit emotional well-being as well as overall health. These benefits are far-reaching and continue long after the meditation session ends.

Diet

A diet high in stress-inducing chemicals, sugars, and refined carbohydrates can negatively affect the adrenal glands, disrupt sleep and hormone function, and adversely influence weight and mood. Stress promotes greater physiological demands, so it's not surprising that we require a more nutrient-dense diet during periods of stress. Ironically, however, stress can cause unhealthy eating habits. When people have chronic stress, they often have little time to fit a balanced diet into their busy schedules. Many individuals turn to fast foods and comfort foods that are high in fat, sugar, and salt and lacking the essential vitamins and minerals their bodies need to deal with stressful circumstances. In addition, when people are stressed or not feeling well, they may skip meals or forget to eat. These dietary insufficiencies can lead to nutritional deficiencies that put an even greater burden on the body, which further compromises metabolic systems and poses a threat to both physical and mental health.

Because people enduring stress are frequently tired, even to the point of exhaustion, they may use coffee or other stimulants to give them a boost of energy and help them cope. But products that contain caffeine, especially in large quantities, can have adverse effects on the body and mind. People who rely on caffeine to stay awake undermine the rest their bodies desperately need and disrupt their natural circadian sleep cycle. Caffeine increases the production of certain hormones in the body, such as adrenaline and cortisol, as well as the neurotransmitter dopamine, which is a precursor of epinephrine. The increased amount of cortisol produced by stress further contributes to the urge to eat foods high in refined carbohydrates, sugars, and fats. Nutritional deficiencies often lead to chronic physical and emotional problems, such as lethargy, lapses in concentration, and mood swings. If the nutritional consequences of stress aren't properly dealt with, the body could suffer serious, long-term health repercussions, such as diabetes, high blood pressure, and high cholesterol.

Although some websites and alternative practitioners specializing in "adrenal fatigue" may advise eating or avoiding certain foods at particular times of the day, there is no scientific evidence to support these suggestions. A special "adrenal fatigue diet" and treatment protocol may help to improve an individual's health, but that's only because it encourages important diet and lifestyle improvements rather than directly providing a boost to adrenal gland function.

Certain whole foods that are naturally high in carbohydrates, such as bananas, brown rice, oatmeal, pumpkins, and sweet potatoes, contain large amounts of tryptophan, an amino acid that helps relax the body and aids sleep. Brown rice, oatmeal, polenta, tart cherries, and walnuts are just some of the many wholesome foods that contain melatonin, the hormone that regulates sleep. Eating a small amount of foods rich in complex carbohydrates a few hours before bedtime will help you fall asleep more quickly and will keep you sleeping more soundly through the night.

All whole-food sources of carbohydrates are also excellent sources of fiber. Fiber regulates digestion, facilitates proper bowel function, and keeps glycemic levels steady so you can stay satisfied longer and won't get hungry quite as quickly. Unlike sugar and caffeine, which cause anxiety and jitteriness, complex carbohydrates provide a grounding effect that reduces anxiety and provides the balance and sustenance your body needs during times of stress. Avoid refined carbohydrates, such as white flour, sugar of any kind (including "healthy" sugars, such as agave nectar, brown rice syrup, brown sugar, honey, maple syrup, and molasses), and breads, rolls, cereals, and other processed foods that contain refined grains or sugars.

Foods That Relieve Stress and Promote Relaxation

Scientists believe that complex carbohydrates cause the brain to produce more serotonin, a hormone that aids relaxation, improves mood, and promotes healthy sleep patterns. High-fiber foods increase satiety, support healthy bowel function, and can help thwart potentially harmful food cravings. Legumes (beans, lentils, peas), oatmeal, sweet potatoes, white potatoes with skin, whole grains (such as brown rice, bulgur, millet, and quinoa), and winter squash are just a few of the foods that fall into this category.

Foods That Exacerbate Stress

Foods that are high in fat, particularly animal fat (such as meat, cheese, and butter), elevate blood pressure, make our blood thick and sticky, and cause us to feel tired and sluggish. As a result, fatty, high-cholesterol foods contribute to weight gain, depression, and lethargy, as well as increase the risk of heart attack.

Although small amounts of caffeine can provide a short-term energy boost and temporarily elevate mood, too much caffeine increases cortisol secretion, raises blood pressure, causes tension and jitteriness, interferes with sleep, and can make people feel stressed even if they weren't to begin with. Drinking caffeinated beverages (coffee, tea, cola) will exacerbate stress, not alleviate it. While it's true that weaning yourself off caffeine can be rough for a few days, it will be beneficial to your long-term stress reduction.

Because sugar is a carbohydrate, it can initially impart a sense of calm. But since it's a simple carbohydrate, it enters and leaves the bloodstream rapidly, causing an energy "rush" followed by a nasty "crash," ultimately creating a vicious up-down cycle that can leave you feeling irritable and drained. It's best to avoid all types of sugar and other simple carbohydrate foods, such as candy, desserts, pastries, sodas, syrups, and white bread.

Many people are under the false impression that alcohol is a relaxant, and they therefore think it's okay to imbibe during periods of stress. While a small glass of wine or a shot of whiskey might provide some short-term relief, in the long run it can do more harm than good. Alcohol damages the liver and depresses adrenal function, and although reduced cortisol production may initially seem like a good thing, over time it can impair the immune system, increase inflammation, and disrupt healthy sleep patterns. To lower stress levels and improve overall health, it's best to avoid alcohol consumption completely.

Culinary Herbs and Spices

Although you're no doubt aware that herbs and spices taste great, you may be surprised to learn that many of them can also help the body cope with acute or chronic stress. In addition, they can help support and strengthen the immune system when the adrenal glands are overwhelmed. Some of the best options are cardamom, cinnamon, cloves, coriander, fennel seeds, garlic, ginger, oregano, peppermint, spearmint, thyme, and turmeric. If you have access to fresh herbs, such as basil, cilantro, dill, mint, oregano, sage, or thyme, all the better. Incorporate these herbs and spices regularly in your meals by adding them to recipes or sprinkling them over finished dishes, whole grains, vegetables, and salads.

Additional Tips

Your body needs fuel at regular intervals throughout the day. Honor that need by giving it real (rather than refined and processed) foods on a consistent basis. Avoid skipping meals, especially breakfast and lunch, as that would result in an unwelcome drop in blood sugar later in the day, along with elevated stress levels.

While it's important to have regularly scheduled meals, monitor your portion sizes. Overeating puts undue stress on the body and slows down digestion, which can make you feel even more sluggish. Eat at a relaxed pace, not on the run or in the car.

Finally, avoid eating right before you go to bed. It takes about three hours for food to be fully processed and digested after you eat, and the body can't properly rest and digest food simultaneously.

Vitamins and Minerals

Poor eating and lifestyle habits as a result of stress can take a terrible toll on nutritional intakes, further burdening the body's systems. When stress overtakes your life, there are a few nutrients in particular that you should pay special attention to. While most of these can be obtained through diet, a few will require supplementation.

B-complex vitamins help with nervous system functioning, and experiencing severe or ongoing stress can deplete your levels. Vitamin B_{12} and other B vitamins play a vital role in producing brain chemicals that affect anxiety and mood and certain brain functions. Low levels of B_{12} and other B vitamins, such as vitamin B_6 and folate, are linked to low energy, fuzzy thinking, poor stress response, and possibly depression. Try to obtain your B vitamins from whole foods (such as almonds, beans, berries, broccoli, dark leafy greens, dried fruits, and fortified nondairy milk and yogurt), but take a B-complex supplement or multivitamin-mineral supplement if you feel your diet is lacking. Almost everyone should supplement with sublingual vitamin B_{12}, which isn't found in sufficient quantities in food to ensure the daily recommended amount. This nutrient is essential to healthy hormones, brain and nervous system function, red blood cell production, and overall health, so supplementing with it, especially for older individuals and anyone under stress, is essential.

Magnesium plays a role in over three hundred of the body's biochemical reactions and regulates the release of stress hormones. Research has shown a strong connection between low magnesium levels and depression and anxiety. Magnesium-rich foods include dark-green leafy vegetables (such as chard, kale, and spinach), as well as avocados, bananas, dark chocolate, figs, legumes (beans, lentils, and peas), nuts (especially almonds, Brazil nuts, and cashews), seeds (especially pumpkin seeds), tofu, and whole grains.

Tryptophan isn't a vitamin or mineral but rather an essential amino acid. It's the leading supplement purchased for stress and anxiety. Tryptophan converts into a compound called 5-HTP, which then converts to serotonin (the "feel good" chemical), which plays an important role in regulating appetite, mood, and sleep. Although all high-protein foods contain tryptophan, that doesn't mean the body can use the tryptophan from those protein sources. For example, cow's milk contains a good amount of tryptophan, but it is also abundant in pro-inflammatory cytokines that will degrade tryptophan. Furthermore, animal-based proteins are loaded with saturated fat and lack fiber and vitamin C, which makes it difficult for the body to use tryptophan for the production of serotonin and melatonin. Surprisingly, some of the best tryptophan-containing foods are plant-based.

Unlike animal products, plants are rich in health-supporting anti-inflammatory fats, fiber, and antioxidants, and many of them also contain the tryptophan cofactors vitamin B_6, vitamin C, folic acid, and magnesium. Good plant-based sources of tryptophan include bananas, dark leafy greens, legumes (beans, lentils, and peas), nuts (especially walnuts), potatoes, seeds (especially pumpkin seeds), soy products (edamame, tempeh, tofu, soy milk), spirulina, whole grains (oats, quinoa, whole wheat), and winter squash.

Vitamin D is known as the "sunshine vitamin" because its main source is sunlight. People who live in climates with cold, dark winters are at significantly higher risk for deficiency, although it's estimated that 30–100 percent of all people are deficient in vitamin D! Research has confirmed that individuals with depression and anxiety disorders commonly have low levels of this nutrient. Fortified foods (such as fortified juices and nondairy milks) may contain a measure of vitamin D, but if you have darker skin, don't spend much time outdoors, or are an older adult, vitamin D supplementation is critical to ensure you're getting adequate amounts.

Calcium deficiency is less common than a deficiency in magnesium, vitamin B_{12}, or vitamin D, but it can nevertheless have a powerful effect on mental and physical health. The nervous system requires calcium to function properly, so mood disorders and anxiety often arise with insufficient calcium intakes. The physical symptoms of calcium deficiency include tingling sensations, numbness, shaking, and heart palpitations, which are also common physical symptoms of anxiety. Calcium-rich food choices include almonds, dark-green leafy vegetables, oatmeal, fortified nondairy milks, and fortified soy products.

Conclusion

If you have been to the doctor for your symptoms, gone through multiple diagnostic tests that have come back negative, and been told there's nothing medically wrong with you, it's time to employ a different strategy. The solution to feeling better is actually close at hand. With the guidance outlined in this book, you can begin to identify the lifestyle patterns and behaviors you're engaging in that are causing your body to be under constant strain and consequently compromising your health. It's crucial to recognize the importance of lifestyle changes that are readily available to you and that can reduce or eliminate your symptoms.

The effects that stress can have on a person's health are serious and can wreak havoc with every major system of the body, resulting in the cluster of symptoms often referred to as "adrenal fatigue." But with the right approaches, you can minimize the impact stress has on your body and effectively repair and reverse any damage that has been done. Wise behavioral choices and a healthy lifestyle are essential companions to any stress-reduction program. The antidote is directly within your reach.

Resources

The American Institute of Stress
stress.org

Cleveland Clinic Center for Continuing Education/Disease Management
clevelandclinicmeded.com

Diet & Fitness Today
dietandfitnesstoday.com

EndocrineWeb
endocrineweb.com

Hormone Health Network
hormone.org

Johns Hopkins Medicine Health Library
hopkinsmedicine.org

Medical News Today
medicalnewstoday.com

Medline Plus
medlineplus.gov

Medscape : Drugs & Diseases
emedicine.medscape.com

National Adrenal Diseases Foundation
nadf.us

The National Center for Biotechnology Information
ncbi.nlm.nih.gov

The National Institute of Diabetes and Digestive and Kidney Diseases
niddk.nih.gov

Pituitary Network Association Knowledge Base
pituitary.org/knowledge-base

Science Daily
sciencedaily.com

Science-Based Medicine
sciencebasedmedicine.org

United States National Library of Medicine, National Institutes of Health
nim.nih.gov

About the Author

Sorrel Davis is a natural-health researcher and has been a longtime advocate of the healing properties of herbal remedies and a proponent of the adage "let food be thy medicine." She is a fan of kite flying, horror films, spicy cuisine, Little League baseball, and dancing as if no one is watching.